MW01244235

A Patient's Guide To Dialysis

by Mike Gurak

Dedication

This book is dedicated to all the men and women who work with dialysis patients, from the doctors to the nurses and techs to... everybody. It is especially dedicated to the men and women of Fresenius Kidney Care Bedford-Blue Ridge and DaVita Peaks of Otter, both of which are in Bedford, VA. Thank you all for making an otherwise scary situation very normal. You don't know how appreciated you are.

Table Of Contents

Introduction

You have just been diagnosed with end stage renal disease (ESRD), or perhaps chronic kidney disease (CKD). Your doctor wants you to start dialysis. A million things are probably going through your head right now. How bad is this going to hurt? Is my life going to revolve around dialysis now? Am I doomed?

I remember thinking all those things. My only experience with dialysis was the 1986 movie *Star Trek IV: The Voyage Home*. In it, an elderly lady is on a gurney moaning. Dr. McCoy asks what's wrong. She answers, "Kidney dialysis." He mutters, "What is this, the Dark Ages?" Not exactly a comforting memory.

But that was over 35 years ago. I don't know what dialysis was like back then but it sure isn't anything like that today. Yes ESRD and CKD are serious. Yes dialysis is serious. But in my opinion dialysis really isn't that bad. It does require a lifestyle adjustment. However it's an adjustment that's very possible to make.

This book doesn't cover ESRD or CKD. There are many good books out there that discuss the diseases. I also don't go into detail about the kidneys, their function, or anything else about them for the same reason.

I do cover the two types of dialysis: hemodialysis and peritoneal dialysis (PD). The first one is the one you're probably familiar with. They put needles in your arm, draw blood out, clean it using a special machine, and put it back in your body. You may not have even heard of the second type. In PD they put a catheter in your abdomen (actually the peritoneum), pump in a special liquid called dialysate, let it sit for a while, then drain it back out.

I also cover the recommended diet for dialysis patients. Not necessarily a menu but more of what not to eat and drink. And most importantly, why.

I also go into some explanation of your care team. These are the folks who will work with you to help you with dialysis and to live the best life you can.

This book is written from my experience. I'm not a medical professional. I'm just a dialysis patient with ESRD. I don't know everything about everything. If you have any questions about something I've talked about, or want information about things I don't cover for whatever reason, talk to your care team. They really are there for you.

So take a few deep breaths and relax. Hopefully I can demystify things for you. And remember: you can do this.

Chapter 1: Hemodialysis

Part 1: About Hemodialysis

In hemodialysis, they put needles in your arm or use a catheter (mine was in my chest), draw out blood, clean it using a special machine, and put it back in you. This happens many times over the course of hours. This chapter is all about hemodialysis, how it works in-center and at home, and a whole host of other things you need to know.

Part 2: In-center Hemodialysis

It's your first day of in-center hemodialysis. Like many (most?) patients your dialysis experience starts here. When you walk through the door they will take your temperature, then you wait to be called back to the dialysis room. Generally visitors aren't allowed in the dialysis room.

There are a number of chairs in the dialysis room. You won't be going through this alone. They will weigh you then bring you back to your chair. They will also check your blood pressure, typically both standing and sitting. In my dialysis center we typically sat in the same row of chairs although the exact chair might vary from day to day.

Then it's time to hook up to the machine. This is done in one of two ways. The most common way is through a fistula in your arm. A fistula is a connection between and artery and a vein. This connection is made in a hospital. The dialysis center staff puts two needles connected to hoses into your fistula.

The other way you can hook up to the machine is through a catheter. This is how I connected. My catheter was placed in my upper right chest. They connect the hoses to the catheter ends.

Once you're connected, they turn on the machine. The machine draws out your blood, filters it, and pumps it back into your body. This is a continuous loop. The staff will check the machine every so often to make sure there aren't any problems.

Many patients typically are in treatment for 4 hours a day, three days a week. Common schedules are Monday, Wednesday, and Friday or Tuesday, Thursday, and Saturday. It generally isn't recommended to have back to back days of hemodialysis although if you need to change a day due to an appointment it can be arranged.

At my dialysis center they took patients in two time slots: 6:00 AM to 10:00 AM and 10:00 AM to 2:00 PM. Typically you will keep the same days and times every week. This makes it very easy and convenient to schedule the rest of your days. This also means that you will see the same patients each time you go in for treatment.

So during treatment you have to sit very still for four hours and watch the time slowly tick by, right? Not at all. You can read as long as you don't do anything that will crimp the hoses or otherwise obstruct the flow of blood. You can do things on your cell phone. My center also provided TVs for patients to watch. Each patient had their own TV. Of course, you need to have headphones. If you forget yours, the center may provide ear buds for you.

Many patients brought in books and blankets. It appears that the body temperature of people with ESRD and CKD is lower than most people's. So a blanket may be helpful. Also, it will help keep you comfortable if you fall asleep during treatment.

That's right, patients actually can fall asleep during treatment. Once they hook you up there's no pain or other discomfort. It simply feels like you're just sitting in a comfy chair for four hours.

The staff set the machines to pull a certain amount of fluid. Usually the nurse will determine the amount, tailored to you and your specific needs. As I mentioned earlier the staff monitors the machines to make sure there are no problems. If there is a problem, the machine emits a tone that alerts staff.

There are two things you as a patient should be on the lookout for. The first is cramping. If you experience cramping anywhere, no matter how minor, let staff know. This generally means they need to allow more liquid into the machine.

The second is feeling dizzy or lightheaded. This usually means your blood pressure is too low. Let staff know right away if you feel this way. In fact, if you feel off in any way, even if it seems inconsequential, let staff know. Especially until you've had a number of treatments and know what to look for. You never know what might signal a problem.

Interesting case in point: early on during hemodialysis I'd get sick to my stomach shortly after my session started. I reported this to the staff. The nurse was able to figure out that I was allergic to the iron they were giving me (I had low iron in my blood). They switched the iron and I was fine from then on.

Depending on your dialysis center, you might or might not be allowed to have a snack during treatment. They usually frown on anything approaching a meal however. Talk to the staff about snacking.

Eventually your treatment time will end for that day. The machine usually emits a special tone to let staff know you're done. Then they will unhook you. If you connected using a fistula, they will wait for the bleeding to stop before you get out of the chair.

They will check your blood pressure again, also typically sitting and standing. Then it's time to get your after treatment weight. That's it. You're done for the day.

Many people, myself included, report feeling tired after hemodialysis. I was exhausted the rest of the day and still somewhat tired the next day. So don't plan on running any marathons after dialysis.

You can travel while on hemodialysis. Let your dialysis center know in plenty of time before you travel so they can find a center in the area you will be in. And of course the staff at the other center will need to arrange days and times for you to get treatment there. Don't walk out the door Friday and tell them you're going out of town tomorrow for a week.

You can travel just about anywhere. Going out of the country may be a problem but otherwise staff should be able to find you a center wherever you're going. So don't let dialysis stop you from visiting relatives and friends or going on that trip you've been planning.

So what about doctor appointments and other obligations that suddenly pop up? Talk to the staff at the center as soon as you know you will need to change the day or time of your treatment for an appointment of other function. They will be happy to work with you. Of course, once you know your regular treatment schedule it's best to make your appointments for other days and times.

Part 3: Hemodialysis At Home

Before I get into hemodialysis at home, let me just say I've never done this. I had someone explain at-home hemodialysis but when I heard about all the advantages of peritoneal dialysis (PD), I chose not to investigate at-home hemodialysis and concentrate solely on PD. So I can only tell you what I was told, not my own experience with it.

You will need to be trained on how to do hemodialysis at home. The dialysis center where you get in-center hemodialysis should be able to train you. I believe it takes 2 to 3 weeks to be fully trained but the staff at the center will explain that to you if and when they offer you the option to do hemodialysis at home.

Unlike peritoneal dialysis, you will need someone with you to do hemodialysis at home. They will be the one to hook you up to the machine. So not only do they have to be able to hook you up and unhook you each time, they must be available for the training the same as you.

Patients generally do hemodialysis at home three or four days a week. I believe dialysis lasts four hours each treatment but again, that's something staff will tell you.

I do know that given the choice between in-center hemodialysis and at-home hemodialysis, at-home is the better way to go for various reasons. One is that it can be done wherever you happen to be. That's typically in the comfort of your own home but it can also be wherever you are if you're traveling.

Part 4: FAQs

Q: Does hemodialysis hurt?

A: Only when they put the needles in and take them out, if you're using a fistula. If you're using a catheter then hooking up and unhooking doesn't hurt. And the actual dialysis process doesn't hurt at all. In fact, a number of patients fall asleep during hemodialysis.

Q: Where can I travel?
A: Generally anywhere in your country. If you're flying, you will probably need something from your doctor saying it's medically necessary for you to travel with your machine. And don't forget to tell your center ahead of time when and where you'll be so they can find a center for you there.

Q: Do I really need a care partner if I'm doing hemodialysis at home? Can't I do it myself?
A: You really do need a care partner. If you don't have anyone who can help you, look into peritoneal dialysis (PD) or simply stay with in-center hemodialysis.

Q: Will I be tired when I do hemodialysis?
A: Yes, probably. Although I understand that patients tend to be less tired doing hemodialysis at home than in-center. This tiredness can last through the next day too.

Q: Can I do hemodialysis three days in a row and get it over with?

A: No. You don't want to go too many days without doing hemodialysis. Generally two days is fine, like the weekends, but anything more than that isn't recommended. The whole point of dialysis is to get rid of the toxins your kidneys can't get rid of on their own. Going too long between sessions can allow these to build up to dangerous levels.

Chapter 2: Peritoneal Dialysis (PD)

Part 1: The Basics

Peritoneal dialysis (PD) is different than hemodialysis. In PD, special liquid called dialysate is pumped into your abdomen (actually your peritoneum), it sits there for a while, then is drained out. When the dialysate is drained it takes with it all the toxins your kidneys can't get rid of on their own.

PD is done at home only. That's one of the great things about PD. You only have to go to the dialysis center twice a month on average: once to get labs drawn and once to meet with your doctor. There are two types of PD. The first used a machine and is generally done at night, often while you sleep. The second is by the manual bag system and can be done anytime.

For PD, a catheter is placed in your abdomen. It's actually in the peritoneum, which is where the name peritoneal dialysis comes from. But most people who aren't familiar with PD will simply be satisfied knowing it's in your abdomen.

The end of the catheter is called the transfer set. This is the end that connects to the hose that goes to the machine, or connects to the bag if you're using the manual bag system. The transfer set should be replaced every six months. Because of the catheter, swimming anywhere other than the ocean or perhaps, if you feel comfortable, a private pool. Public pools and other swimming places are extremely not recommended due to the potential bacteria.

It generally takes eight to ten days of around four hours a day to learn how to do PD. Your hemodialysis center may also teach PD, or as in my case you may have to switch to a new center. You will need to have a care partner learn along with you although when you actually do PD at home you can do it all alone.

PD has a few benefits over hemodialysis. The first is it doesn't use your blood. The second is many patients report they're not nearly as tired on PD as with hemodialysis. The third is you have more of your day to yourself, even if you use the manual bag system. Of course, if you use the machine method it's done while you sleep so the day is yours to do with whatever you want. I understand that for these and other reasons doctors are having more and more patients do PD over hemodialysis.

Part 2: PD Using The Machine

The machine used for PD is called a cycler. It's my understanding that most people who do PD do so with the cycler although some prefer the manual bag system.

PD using the cycler starts by gathering your supplies. The first thing you will need is the dialysate. It comes in three different strengths, each of which has a different color code. The first is 1.5% solution which is yellow. (The colors are the colors of the tape used to seal the box and the plugs at the end of the bags. Your solution should be clear.) The second is 2.5% solution which is green. The third is 4.24% solution which is red.

Although dialysate comes in a number of different volumes, for PD using the machine you will generally use either 5,000ml (5 liter) bags or 6,000ml (6 liter) bags. At first you will probably only use two bags per night, although later some people use three.

Be sure to warm the dialysate on the cycler before you use it. When you train on doing PD they will tell you the range of temperatures the dialysate should be between. They should also tell you how long to leave the bags on the cycler to get them to the proper temperature. **Do not** use dialysate that hasn't been warmed to this temperature.

The second thing you will need is the cassette. This is the "set" the cycler will tell you to load. It has a drain line of approximately twenty feet, so if your bedroom is near the bathroom you can place it in the tub or in the sink. It also has a patient line of about twenty feet. This gives you enough room to walk around a small one bedroom apartment like I do. You are tethered to the cycler to a degree but you don't have to stay right next to it. You can sit in a chair in your bedroom or another room if it's close enough.

You will need a mini cap to put on the end of the transfer set when your treatment is finished. You use Exsept to clean the exit site of your catheter and Alcavis to clean the transfer set. Both of these will help prevent peritonitis, which is a nasty infection of the peritoneum. Finally you will need a lap pad (one of those blue plastic and cloth things they use in doctor's offices and hospitals to put their instruments on to keep them sterile), assorted gauze pads, and some tape.

Before you start PD you need to weigh yourself and record the weight. Then you need to do the same with your blood pressure and pulse. Depending on your dialysis center you may need to check your temperature as well.

Now you're ready to start dialysis. Basically you put the cassette in the cycler, hook up the bags of dialysate, then hook yourself to the machine. Be sure to follow all the steps exactly and carefully, just like you were taught at the center. Once the machine says "fill 1 of X" (where X is the number of fills for the night), you're good to go. You can go right to bed if you want or you can stay up. It's your choice.

Usually dialysis takes around eight hours. Many patients have either three or four fills for the night of around 2,500ml each. So you're probably looking at 7,500ml or 10,000ml a night. That's why dialysate comes in 5,000ml and 6,000ml bags.

There are three phases to a fill: the actual fill of about 15 minutes where the cycler pumps the dialysate into your peritoneum, a dwell phase of typically one and a half to two hours or so where the dialysate sits in you and does its work, and the drain phase which is about another 15 minutes.

When dialysis is over, the machine will say "end of treatment". Just like when you hooked up to the machine, follow all the steps exactly and carefully to unhook. And don't forget to have the cycler do a manual drain. It normally won't drain all the dialysate by itself without it.

Part 3: PD Using The Manual Bag System

The manual bag system is a alternative to using the cycler. Most patients, from what I understand, use the cycler. So why use the manual bag system?

Quite simply, because sometimes you have to. The cycler runs on electricity. If that goes out, you need the bag system. I'll also use it if I'm afraid the power will go out during the night. Some particularly bad storms, both windstorms and thunderstorms, have been known to knock out the power for hours at a time. It's great as a backup.

I will admit however that I'm not quite as well versed on the bag system and I am using the cycler. I had one (or maybe a half?) day of training on the bag system compared to seven (and a half?) days with the cycler. So all I can tell you is how I do things. Definitely check with your dialysis center if you have any questions.

Just like with the cycler, using the manual bag system starts with gathering your supplies. You won't need the cassette but you will need two clamps, one for the fill line and one for the drain line. You will need all the other supplies as wen you use the cycler. The bags for the manual bag system generally come in 2,000ml volumes and are used only one bag at a time. Don't forget your IV pole. Most people do the bag system three to five times a day. I like to let the dialysate dwell for three to three and a half hours but definitely talk to the staff at your dialysis center for their recommendation. You will need to warm the dialysate up, just like when you use the cycler. How you do that when the power is out is something to, you guessed it, talk to the staff about.

You will need to record your weight, blood pressure, pulse, and possible your temperature. The bag system has three phases to each fill cycle, just like the cycler. The only difference is gravity does all the work here. Follow all the steps exactly and carefully to start and end each fill cycle. During the dwell phase you are free to go anywhere and do anything. Just be back in time for the drain cycle.

Part 4: Traveling With PD

Just like with hemodialysis you are free to travel while on PD. In fact in some ways traveling with PD is even easier. You still need to find a dialysis center where you will be but you will only need them in an emergency.

If you're traveling by car you will need to pack your machine. I typically bring my own dialysate and all my supplies. But you could have dialysate shipped to wherever you're going.

If you're traveling by plane you will need to bring your machine too. You will probably need something from your doctor explaining that it is medically necessary to have the machine. You can have your dialysate delivered to wherever you're going. You will need to bring your other supplies though.

Of course, if you do the manual bag system you can have your dialysate delivered or bring it with you. You will need to pack all of your other supplies. And don't forget to bring the IV pole.

Part 5: FAQs

Q: Does PD hurt?
A: Not at all. If it hurts, contact the nurse at your dialysis center.

Q: Where can I travel?
A: Generally anywhere in your country. If you're flying, you will probably need something from your doctor saying it's medically necessary for you to travel with your machine. And don't forget to tell your center ahead of time when and where you'll be so they can find a center for you there.

Q: Do I really need a care partner?
A: While you're training, yes you do. Someone else needs to know how to do this too. At home, no you don't. You can do it all alone, like I do. That's one of the benefits of PD.

Q: How many days a week do I need to do PD?
A: Short answer, as many as your doctor tells you. You will typically start out doing it every day. Me, I do it five days a week but that's because my doctor said I only need to do it that often. Please don't skip any days.

Q: Will I be tired on PD?
A: It's possible but most people aren't nearly as tired on PD as they are on hemodialysis. You should hopefully see a increase in your energy levels.

Q: Isn't it hard to sleep with PD?
A: That depends on the person. Some people sleep just fine. Me, I don't sleep as well on nights when I do PD. You might not have any trouble.

Chapter 3: Your Care Team

Part 1: Overview

Your care team is a very big part of your dialysis experience. They really are there to help you through this time and to make sure you have the best experience possible. If you have any questions about anything, ask the appropriate member of your care team. Trust me, if they don't know the answer they'll find out.

Your care team consists of the following people: your nephrologist, your nurse (possibly two nurses with in-center hemodialysis), your dietitian, your social worker, and for in-center hemodialysis a few technicians. (My apologies if that's not what they're called.) I'll go into detail about each one.

Part 2: Your Nephrologist

Your nephrologist is your kidney doctor. (The person who reads the bumps on your head is a phrenologist. I know, they sound similar.) This is the big boss on your care team. They decide your treatment plan, from how long to be on dialysis for hemodialysis to what strength dialysate to use for PD to what medicines you should be on.

For in-center hemodialysis you will probably see either the nephrologist or a PA once a week. For PD you will probably see them once a month. I don't know how often you see them on at-home hemodialysis.

Which type of dialysis you are doing will determine what your nephrologist needs to do for you. They will always review your labs and make both medicine and treatment adjustments based on them. If you have any questions about your treatment, medicine, or your kidneys in general this is the person to talk to.

Part 3: Your Nurse(s)

As important as your nephrologist is, you will probably have more contact with the nurse(s). I say nurses plural because in my experience, in in-center hemodialysis there is a head nurse and typically a second nurse on duty as well. You will see a nurse every time you do hemodialysis.

For PD, and quite possibly at-home hemodialysis, you will see the nurse twice a month. The first time they will draw your labs and do some quick educating. The second time you see them is when you also see your nephrologist. They will tell your doctor what's been going on since the last doctor visit.

They are also the person you will contact if you have any questions or run into any problems.

Part 4: Your Dietitian

Your dietitian is a good source of information about what to eat and drink to stay healthy with ESRD or CKD while on dialysis. This is generally the person who will talk to you about your lab results in-depth and make any suggestions on how to bring your numbers up or lower them as needed. How often you see your dietitian depends on what kind of dialysis you're doing and how often you have labs drawn.

Be sure your dietitian knows about any co-occurring conditions you have, such as diabetes that also require a special diet. If you have any diet related questions, this is the person to talk to.

Part 5: Your Social Worker

Whether you are doing in-center hemodialysis, at-home dialysis, or PD you will have a social worker. They are a great source of information on all kinds of resources. They will help make sure you have everything you need. This may be the first time you have had a social worker. Don't be afraid to ask them what they can and can't help you with.

Part 6: Your Techs

In my experience you will only see techs when you do in-center hemodialysis. They are just like the techs in a hospital. These are the folks who are most often working the dialysis machines. When the machines emit a warning tone thy are usually the people who respond. They help the nurses with the day to day operations.

Chapter 4: Your New Diet

Part 1: An Overview

Just like any other disease or condition, having ESRD or CKD means having a new diet. There are some things you shouldn't have, some you should only eat or drink occasionally, and some things you can either have or are encouraged to have.

The problem with ESRD and CKD of course is your kidneys can't get rid of some of the toxins your body produces. That's why you're on dialysis. Some foods and drinks contain things that will build up in your body. These are things you should either avoid or eat or drink sparingly.

Interestingly, you are more restricted with in-center hemodialysis than on PD. (I don't know about at-home hemodialysis.) There are a few reasons for this. The first is simply that you do PD every day (or nearly every day, as in my case). The second is you are doing PD for longer each day than hemodialysis. This is just another benefit of being on PD.

There are a few things to watch out for. The big two are potassium and phosphorus. Your dietitian will give you a list of everything to watch out for but here I'll cover potassium and phosphorus. You may never have had to watch out for these two before so that's why I'm giving them special attention.

Part 2: Potassium

Potassium is easy to spot on food labels. If it lists "potassium {something}" it has potassium in it. Simple, right? But did you know that potatoes, tomatoes, and bananas have a lot of potassium in them as well?

If you can help it, avoid foods with potassium, or at least choose foods that are low in potassium. If you're on hemodialysis it's probably best to avoid those fries, tomatoes including pizza sauce, and bananas. Other foods have natural potassium in them as well. Your dietitian should give you a fairly lengthy list of them and suggest good alternatives.

Again, if you're on PD you don't have to worry **quite** as much. But I still wouldn't recommend getting a medium fry from a fast food restaurant.

Having too much potassium in your system can be dangerous or even deadly. It can lead to irregular heartbeat, muscle weakness, a weak or irregular pulse, and heart palpitations, among other things.

Part 3: Phosphorus

Phosphorus is a little harder to find on food labels. Unlike potassium it won't be listed as "phosphorus {something}". It will be listed as "phos{something}". If you see "phos" at the start of an ingredient, it's probably best to avoid it all together.

One of the big culprits is actually dark sodas. It's best to avoid the colas and go with a lemon lime soda. Interestingly enough, root beer is fine.

One other food that might surprise you is lunch meat. I've given it up completely and my numbers reflect that. Sigh, and I love my ham and cheese sandwiches.

High phosphorus levels can lead to heart attacks or strokes, weak bones (it pulls the calcium out of them), and some other nasty things. It's best to keep your phosphorus in the levels your doctor recommends.

Part 4: Fluid Restrictions

One of the things typically associated with ESRD, and possibly CKD, is decreased urine output. Put another way, you pee less. So liquid builds up in your system. Obviously this isn't good for you. Your body needs to maintain a balance.

So not surprisingly dialysis patients often have fluid restrictions. It's not a matter of what you drink, although see the above parts on potassium and especially phosphorus, but how much you drink. 32 ounces of liquid a day seems to be normal, although your doctor can vary this to meet your own circumstances. For example, at first I was limited to 50 ounces a day, especially when I was on hemodialysis. Now though I make enough urine that I'm not currently restricted. I also know someone who was limited to either 2 or 4 ounces of liquid a day, just enough to take her pills with.

It's up to you how much you drink when as long as you stay within that limit. For example, if you're limited to 32 ounces a day you could have 8 ounces each with breakfast, lunch, and dinner and 8 ounces at bedtime. Or you could drink a liter of soda with lunch and that's all the liquid you get that day. Be aware that the milk in your cereal and the liquid in soup counts towards your daily limit.

Chapter 5: My Story

Before I wrap up this book I wanted to share with you my experiences with ESRD and dialysis. My story isn't exactly typical (you'll see why) but it's one story among millions. Hopefully you'll get something out of it. Honestly, I think sharing my story and writing this book are the reason why I have ESRD and am on dialysis.

Back in December 2021 I had a sore on my right foot. It had gotten infected so I went to the ER. I knew they would keep me for a few days. While I was there they discovered that my creatine level, which is an indicator of how well your kidneys are functioning, was extremely high. It should be a 1. Mine was an 8. They were able to get it down to a 2 so they released me on Christmas Eve, after 10 days in the hospital.

Things were going along alright for a short while. I started coughing at night. Sleeping in my recliner helped. Then one night I had a hard time breathing. The visiting nurse who was taking care of my foot checked my oxygen. It was 75%. It should be in the very high 90s. This was January 3, 2022. I had been home only 10 days.

She called the ambulance and they brought me to the hospital. On the way I almost couldn't breathe. They put me on oxygen. I didn't get off the oxygen for months.

While I was in the hospital they found out that my creatine level was back up to 8. They couldn't get it back down so they decided to start dialysis in the hospital. They couldn't get anything in my veins so they had to put a catheter in my chest. Eventually I ended up in the ICU. I was so bad off they called my family and said it would be a good time to say their goodbyes just in case.

Fortunately I started to recover and they released me after three weeks. I was in rehab for two weeks. The whole time I was on dialysis and oxygen. While I was in rehab I started in-center hemodialysis.

I had no idea what to expect. What would happen here? Sure I had dialysis in the hospital but I was lying in a bed. How would things be different now?

Before that the only thing I knew about dialysis was from *Star Trek IV: The Voyage Home*. Was I going to be like that lady? In a whole lot of pain and going through who knew what? And what did Dr. McCoy mean about were they in the Dark Ages? Just how bad was dialysis anyway?

Of course, that was over 35 years before. Who knew how things had changed. The one thing that struck me about dialysis was how normal everybody made it seem. I liked being with the same people, both staff and patients, each time. And being able to watch TV the whole four hours I was in the chair wasn't so bad. Mind you, I had gotten out of the habit of watching network TV.

After I was released from rehab I went to a dialysis center just down the road from me. Here too I got to know the staff and the other patients. My creatine level kept slowly coming down. Things were looking up but I was hardly out of the woods.

After a few months my nephrologist had to make the call whether I had CKD, ESRD, or would recover. He decided that I did in fact have ESRD. One of the first things they did after that was start talking to me about either doing hemodialysis at home or doing PD. I quickly decided that PD was the route I wanted to go. I hate needles. If I could avoid them and avoid getting a fistula, that would be great. Besides, I live alone. I didn't have anyone who could help me with at-home hemodialysis three or four days a week. PD I could do on my own once my training was done.

Besides, PD offered me some advantages I couldn't pass up. I would most likely be a lot less tired. I wouldn't be as restricted in my diet. And having to eat a diabetic diet anyway, that sounded good. Plus there were other advantages. I was sold.

I remember going to have my PD catheter put in. They told me that the first day I would have some pain, a lot of pain the second day, a little the third, then no pain after that. They were right. Unfortunately the pharmacy I was using screwed up on the prescription for my pain medication. I had to go to a different pharmacy. So I wasn't on anything for pain until the middle of the second day. I highly recommend getting the pain medication as quickly as possible.

I couldn't use my catheter right away. I had to let it heal for about two weeks. But finally I was able to transfer to a dialysis center that did PD. My old center did at-home hemodialysis but not PD. I trained for four days, four hours a day. I started on a Monday. That Friday and the next Monday I had to do in-center hemodialysis. Because I wasn't getting full sessions of PD, my nephrologist thought this was the best thing for me. Tuesday I was back to PD training and finished on Friday.

My dialysis supplies had come in that week so I was almost all set. When I got home that Friday the nurse dropped off my cycler and did a quick home inspection to make sure everything was OK.

This was in August of 2022. Just a few months later I was doing so well my doctor changed my schedule so I only had to do PD five days a week. He suggested I take off Tuesdays and Thursdays. Thursday worked well for me but I decided to take off Saturdays since I have church on Sundays. This was I could go to the earlier Mass if I wanted to or needed to.

I'm also only doing three fills a night. When I started PD I was doing four. And I'm still using yellows (the dialysate) which is not only the lowest strength but the strength I started with.

As I write this I've been on PD for almost a year. Going with PD was the best decision for me. I've done a little traveling and brought my cycler and supplies with me. I love not having to go to the center to do dialysis. I enjoy having my days free to do whatever I want. And I love that I can do PD on my own.

There is a downside to it though. I don't sleep well on the nights I do PD. I think I'm subconsciously aware of the tube connected to my catheter, even while I sleep. And when my cycler gets to the drain cycle I usually have to be on my right side or I'll get a "low drain volume" warning. Man that beeping is annoying. I have it on the lowest volume but it still wakes me out of a sound sleep, as it should.

So that's my story. In some ways it's my own. In many ways though it's similar to many people's story.

Chapter 6: In Conclusion

Dialysis can be a real Godsend for people with CKD or ESRD. With three different types of dialysis to choose from there's bound to be one that will fit your lifestyle.

And that's the thing. You can have a life. You may even have a long and happy life. Things don't have to come to a complete standstill just because of ESRD or CKD and dialysis. Go where you want, do what you want, live your life.

One thing I haven't covered here is kidney transplantation. That would be a whole other book, one I may write someday. Know though that depending on your situation it may be a possibility.

One final note: this is a life changing disease. It will have an impact on you. Don't be afraid to seek therapy if you need it. If you don't have a therapist, talk to your social worker. They should know of some great places to get the help you need.

Glossary

CKD: Chronic kidney disease. A discussion of CKD is outside this book. There are many good resources for learning about CKD.

dialysate: The liquid used in **peritoneal dialysis**. It comes in three strengths and a number of different amounts.

dialysis: A process by which the toxins that are normally removed by the kidneys are removed from the patient. See **hemodialysis** and **peritoneal dialysis**.

dwell: One of three parts of the fill phase of **peritoneal dialysis**. This is when the **dialysate** is allowed to rest in the patient's body for a period of time.

ESRD: End stage renal disease. A discussion of ESRD is outside this book. There are many good resources for learning about ESRD.

fistula: A connection made between an artery and a vein. Many patients on **hemodialysis** have a fistula surgically created. This is where the needles enter the patient's body.

green(s): The medium strength **dialysate** solution, at 2.5% The color refers to the color of the plug in the dialysate bag and the tape used to seal the carton the bags come in.

hemodialysis: One of two types of dialysis. In hemodialysis blood is drawn from the patient, cleaned in a special machine, and put back in the patient.

nephrologist: A kidney doctor. A nephrologist is one member of a patient's care team.

PD: Short for peritoneal dialysis.

peritoneal dialysis: One of two types of dialysis. In peritoneal dialysis (PD) special liquid called dialysate is pumped into the abdomen (peritoneum), sits for a period of time, and is drawn back out.

red(s): The highest strength **dialysate** solution, at 4.25%. The color refers to the color of the plug in the dialysate bag and the tape used to seal the carton the bags come in.

transfer set: The end of the PD catheter that connects to the cycler

yellow(s): The lowest strength **dialysate** solution, at 1.5%. The color refers to the color of the plug in the dialysate bag and the tape used to seal the carton the bags come in.

About The Author

Mike Gurak lives in Bedford, Virginia, the home of the National D-Day Memorial. Born and raised in New York State, he moved to Virginia when he was 39. He now considers Bedford his home.

Mike writes poems, short stories, and the occasional song. He loves to sing and is a cantor at church. Mike is the eldest of 5 children. His mother, Betty Gurak, wrote a book titled *The Cycle of Grief*, available from Amazon.

This is Mike's fourth book. He also wrote *Let Me Tell You A Story*, a book of short stories and witticisms, a book of poetry titled *My Heart In Twenty-Four Lines*, and *Say What Now?*, a book of misquotes and misattributed quotes. All three books are available as Kindle books from Amazon.

Made in the USA
Middletown, DE
04 November 2023

41840502R00027